AXIOMS
FOR SURVIVORS

———

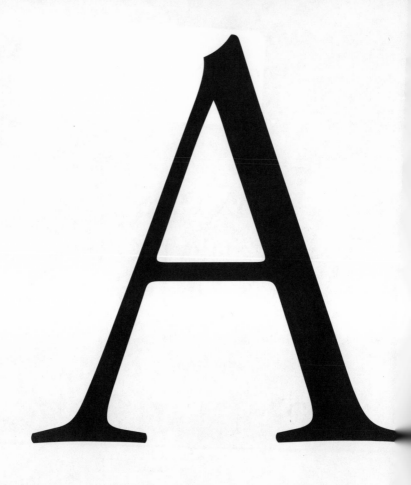

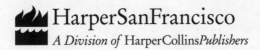

HarperSanFrancisco
A Division of HarperCollins*Publishers*

Lon G. Nungesser

XIOMS

FOR SURVIVORS

—

How to Live
Until You Say Goodbye

FIRST HARPERCOLLINS EDITION PUBLISHED IN 1992.

TEXT DESIGN & ILLUSTRATION BY IRENE IMFELD

Library of Congress Cataloging-in-Publication Data
Nungesser, Lon G.
    Axioms for survivors : how to live until you say goodbye /
Lon G. Nungesser.—Expanded ed.
        p.   cm.
    ISBN 0-06-250698-6 (pbk. : alk. paper)
    1. Consolation—Quotations, maxims, etc.   2. Chronically
ill—Quotations.   I. Title.
BV4910.N86   1992
155.9'16—dc20   91–59052
                                                                  CIP

---

92 93 94 95 96 ❖ FAIR 10 9 8 7 6 5 4 3 2 1

This edition is printed on acid-free paper that meets the American National Standards Institute Z39.48 Standard.

To my friends
with love and
passion for life.

Foreword

Several years ago Lon Nungesser and I crossed paths. We met because Lon was confronting a serious illness while I was trying to teach people in Lon's situation about survival.

Lon has not only become a survivor, but a teacher as well. I respect his courage and have learned from his experience. Lon's life and his book teach us what survival is all about. It is not about living forever; more importantly, it is about living now.

There are some who are not afraid to confront adversity, people who find within themselves the mental and physical resources required to challenge life and to survive. When these special individuals are able to share their wisdom they become healers and teachers for us all. This book contains a wisdom that can guide you on your unique path of healing.

Inside of each of us there is a wisdom that knows the way. You don't have to lead a horse home. The horse knows the way. Some of us have the courage to seek our true path through the darkness rather than the path others create or put us on. I believe Lon's axioms can act as signposts through this uncharted territory. There is an incredible amount of information condensed into these axioms. One need not be sick to benefit from them, only alive and willing to challenge life.

When I read Lon's axioms I find myself nodding, yes! I know the problems with which we are normally confronted and the fears accompanying physical illness. At these times we need a teacher.

It would be nice if we were each born with a manual on how to live, or were taught how to do so early in life by experts. Until such a miracle occurs, we have a good start in these axioms. Read them, learn from them, and let them become a part of your consciousness. I like to read one every morning to start my day with a sense of focus and control.

Axioms for Survivors provides a kind of group therapy. When you sit in a room with others who share similar problems, you learn from each other. When you cannot be in such a group, try the axioms. Their simple, native wisdom here will guide you, confront you, and support you. Remember, the lesson isn't how not to die, but how to *live*—and make of your life a bright torch lighting the way, for yourself, and those you love.

Bernie Siegel, M.D.

AXIOMS
FOR SURVIVORS

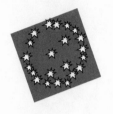

An Event to Be Adapted To

News of a life-threatening illness is an event to be adapted to, not a death sentence to be compliant with.

The Power of Private Prayer

Pray to the God with whom you have sought
and found peace.

Stigma

Much of the initial impact of any diagnosis will be due to the stigma attached to the illness.

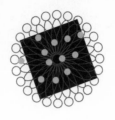

Initial Reaction to Diagnosis

Your initial reaction can make the difference between taking charge of your living or giving in to dying.

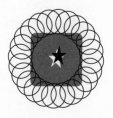

Guarding Against Bad Influences

Be especially careful in selecting the first person you tell about your illness. This person's beliefs about you and your illness may influence you in ways for which you aren't prepared.

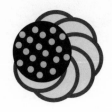

Confidentiality

Make sure you are comfortable in the company of the person you tell first about your illness.

Ask yourself, "Can this person realistically keep my news confidential for the period of time I need?"

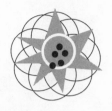

Give-up-itus Is Catching

After you learn that you have a life-threatening illness, take care in whom you choose to tell about your illness. Choose only those people who are confident in your ability to deal with crises. Will they be the kind of person to encourage you not to give up?

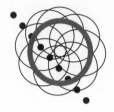

Good Support People

A good support person is the kind of person who can help both you and the other people you will want to tell about your illness.

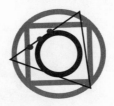

Don't Dwell on Negative Thoughts

When your mind wanders back to the question What did I do to deserve this illness? say aloud to yourself, "Don't dwell!"

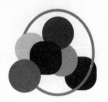

Satisfaction Through Communication

The key to creating satisfaction in your life is in an open and direct manner of communicating with others.

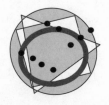

People and Groups
That Support You

Talking with others who are going through
what you are can help you to learn about the
seemingly uncharted territory ahead of you.

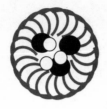

Getting Out of Unhappy Ruts

Don't let yourself get into a rut that reflects
either an I-don't-deserve-to-be-happy or an
I-should-not-be-happy attitude.

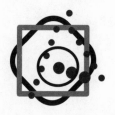

The Power of Simple Distraction

You may find it helpful to simply distract yourself sometimes with a healthy activity you enjoy, like going to a movie, walking in the park, or taking a hot bath.

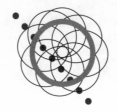

It Is Never Too Late for Prevention

It is never too late for prevention. Make each moment of your life geared toward minimizing illness and maximizing healthful, happy feelings.

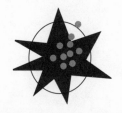

Taking Charge of
Medical Treatments

Taking charge of your medical treatment is
a major part of moving from the dread of diagnosis to empowerment over it.

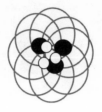

Treatment Options

When a doctor gives you several treatment options, make a mental note, or better still, a written note, on how the doctor presented it to you.

Was it in terms of your survival if you do the treatment versus your death if you don't? If so, beware of this kind of medical manipulation.

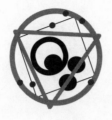

Either/Or Versus Both/And

When making decisions about medical care, try to avoid the trap of thinking you have to choose from either this or that; adopt the attitude that you can select from both this and that.

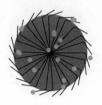

Know What's Going On with Your Body

A very practical way to know what is going on with your body is to always request a copy of your routine blood tests and keep them in a binder.

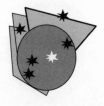

Separation Anxiety and Self-Care

You may feel lost at first if you decide not to consult a doctor for every little thing that appears problematic. Get a good medical dictionary, *The Merck Manual of Diagnosis and Therapy*, and the *Physician's Desk Reference* to ease this loss.

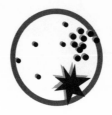

Weigh the Risks and Benefits

Do not take any prescription or nonprescription drugs that will worsen your medical condition. Avoid activities or relationships that damage your body or further the disease process. Try always to weigh the risks and the benefits of all your decisions before you act on them.

Early Warning Signs

Ask your primary care provider to help you compile a list of symptoms and bodily functions to watch for as early warning signs of conditions that require immediate medical attention.

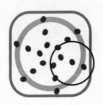

Intervening Thoughts

If you are thinking, *I deserve to die for all the things I have done,* stop that thought! Replace it with, *I may have behaved in ways that damaged my health in the past, but I now have the time and desire to do things differently.*

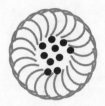

Good Things You Have Done

Recall some of the good things you have done that a person who may "deserve" to die just could not have done. Make an "early career achievements" list, for example. Or list the thoughtful things you have done to help others.

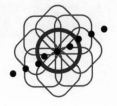

Patience with Others

Be patient with your friends and loved ones as they come to terms with their own reactions to your illness.

Deserved Respect

Remind yourself that you do deserve to be
treated with courtesy and respect.

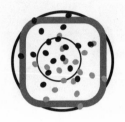

Challenging Blame

Protecting the integrity of your character from social assassination will require you to challenge attitudes that blame and punish you for your illness.

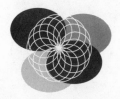

Your Behavior or Your Character

When you are confronted about what led you to become ill, consider if it was a behavior that could have been changed before you seek to blame your character.

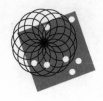

Influencing the Outcome

Ignoring your feelings can have a negative impact on your physical health. You must get in touch with yourself if you hope to effectively influence the outcome of your illness.

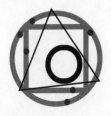

Gaining Self-Acceptance
and Clarity

You can gain self-acceptance and clarity of
mind by knowing what you are feeling most
of the time.

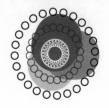

Bound to Controllable Circumstance

Your emotional state is often bound to external situations and events. Therefore, you can get a grip on your situation rather than participating in your own victimization.

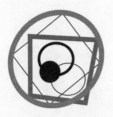

Expressing Your Feelings

Expressing your feelings about what is happening to your health and to your living situation can help you to grow beyond these seemingly limiting circumstances.

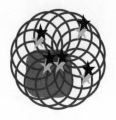

Safe Place to Express Yourself

It is critical that you have a nonjudgmental place where you can express your feelings about what is happening in your life. This place should make you feel safe.

Redefining Loss As Challenge

You may be surprised, but you might gain
some positive things from being ill. One of
the best ways to realize these gains is to
redefine situations or events that seem like a
loss, as a challenge.

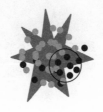

Setting Up Success

Set moderately high goals that you can achieve one at a time. Set up a guaranteed success!

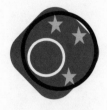

Realizing Goals

When you want to achieve something, break down your long-range goal into sub-goals that can be attained in the short term. Considering the specific steps and means makes it easier to reach the goal.

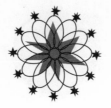

Choose Your Contacts Carefully

You will need to develop a quality of social support that you are satisfied with. Take the time to think through just what you need from others, then choose only to be with the people who meet your values and needs.

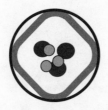

Taking Stock of Past Relationships

Taking stock of your past relationships will help guide you in developing the relationships you need now.

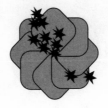

Tough People Need Love, Too

Be persistent and self-confident under the pressure of a life-threatening illness. But, also remind your loved ones that you still need support.

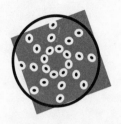

Out of Hiding into the Future

You don't have to be a person who lives in the past, hiding from the possibilities of the future.

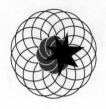

Faith Healing

To many people, hope in the face of a seemingly hopeless situation is acceptable if it is based in religious faith and the grace of God. Be careful. Faith healing can be fatal.

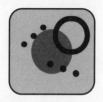

Active Faith Restores Hope

There are many ways for active faith to re-store hope—a hope that rejects death as an evil end to life. I planted garden vegetables that would take longer to harvest than I was supposed to live, and I lived to eat them, too!

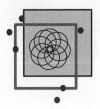

Living Goals

Set specific goals that keep you connected
to the living.

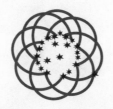

Brains and Willpower

I have seen too many friends die who believed in a judgmental God, but not enough in themselves to promote their own well-being. Why do you think God gave us brains and willpower?

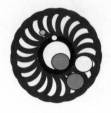

Be Gentle with Yourself

If you experience difficulty in persuading yourself to change your expectations from negative to positive, be gentle with yourself. Be your own best friend. Take the time to place your hands over your heart and quietly say to yourself, "I love you."

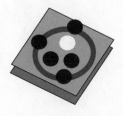

True Failure

Confront the possibility of death openly.
Death is not failure. Living under the excuse
of self-imposed limitations, however, might
be considered failure.

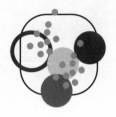

Appreciating Life

One of the most important feelings to have is a satisfaction with life. Those who appreciate the value their life has to themselves and to others, enjoy life more. Recognizing that your life has meaning and that you make a difference can help lessen your anxiety about death.

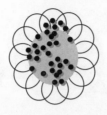

Death Is Not Surrender

I do not feel that to accept death is to surrender. Hope in the face of death is not denial.

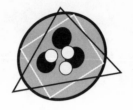

Hope and Resilience

Hope is an important element of survival. Hope can be learned from past experiences.

Recollect successes you have had in the face of obstacles. Make a list of the toughest times in your life and your ways of coping effectively.

Maybe obstacles are placed in our path to make us more resilient . . .

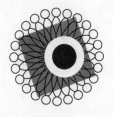

History of Mastery

I have mastered difficult situations before.

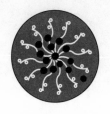

Lifting Yourself Up
by the Bootstraps

I know I am a good person, that I deserve to live, and that I am strong enough to get through today.

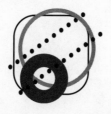

Finding a Sense of Purpose

The connection that you have to your career and to the material world does not diminish readily. Ask yourself, "What gives me a sense of purpose?", then list as many options as you can think of that would fulfill your needs.

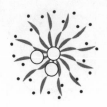

Your Self-Worth to Others

A critical first step in meeting your respon-
sibilities to friends is to hold on to your sense
of self-worth. Consider how you want to be
thought of, the images you want your name
to draw forth. The message you will impart
to your loved ones by dying with your self-
esteem intact will leave them facing life
courageously.

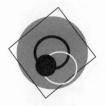

Self-Knowledge

If others think me unfriendly, I can remember that I am a friendly, generous, and thought-ful person, when I am feeling better.

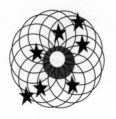

Your Self-Respect

I do not deserve ill treatment from any person.

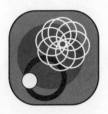

Your Personal Power

I am not helpless, and I do not have to be alone.

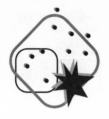

Fighting Effectively

I am learning how to be an effective fighter.

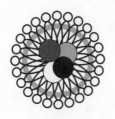

Bladder Theory of Emotions

I have never liked the "bladder theory of emotions" approach to handling feelings, in which you let things build up and, once your feelings are released, you are fine. Rather, it is in the daily process of experiencing heartfelt emotions and finding appropriate ways to express them that makes living both a relief and a pleasure.

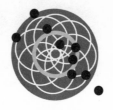

Anger and Tears for Mutual Loss

Anger that loved ones feel toward the person facing a life-threatening illness is often very appropriate. Spend some time with yourself to come to terms with the anger you may experience from others. Allow loved ones to be angry at you for leaving them. Then cry with them about the mutual loss.

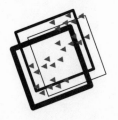

The Grief in My Mother's Eyes

A hospice social worker once said to me that death was much harder on the living than on the dying. I wanted to punch him until I let my heart see the grief in my mother's eyes.

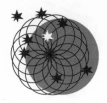

The Love of Friends and Family

The greatest challenge of each moment is to let your very soul experience the love around you. Go beyond the pain of fearing loss to the joy that exists only in the love of your friends and family.

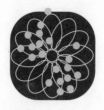

Turning On the Soul Light

A friend of nearly twenty years told me of his experiences with losing many friends to death since we last met. He was stronger than I ever imagined him to be. When I queried him on his newfound inner strength, he said, "I've learned how to help others turn on their soul light and seize each moment."

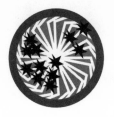

Fear of Being Left Behind

You may be given more advice and direction about your treatment and care than you would like to hear. When this happens, try to understand that the greater motive for such concern often comes from the other person's fear of being left behind.

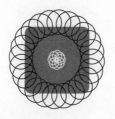

Creating a Meaningful Life

Find the reasons that make life worth living
and you create a meaningful life.

Fear Serves Its Purpose

Fear serves its purpose. Fear provides a fertile environment for divine courage and spiritual growth.

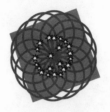

Seeing Who You Really Are

Fear is often the stimulus that causes us to look beyond who we thought we were to see who we really are.

Advice from Your Heart

The best advice you will ever receive will come from your own heart.

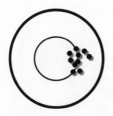

Never Doubt Yourself

Doubting those you love and trust after receiving news of a life-threatening illness is a normal reaction when your world is turned inside out. But doubting yourself after receiving such news must not be indulged in.

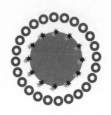

Expect a Masterpiece

When you mix your love and your skills in your recipe for living, don't just expect a miracle—expect a masterpiece!

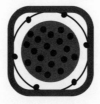

The Rewards of Self-Honesty

What you become by staying true to yourself will be much greater than any material rewards.

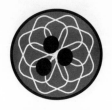

Loving Others

Loving your friends demands your emotions, intellect, soul, and manners—your whole self. Only then are you worthy of them.

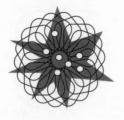

Permission to Feel Bad

Feeling bad is just one part of life. I don't always tell myself I mustn't feel bad. Some days I tell myself, "I think, today, I'll really feel bad!"

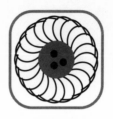

Happiness

You may find yourself surprised one morning by a feeling you do not recognize; somehow, through all the fear and grieving, up has popped happiness!

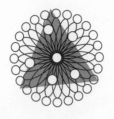

Saving Time on Chitchat

I know of a kindergarten teacher who has a figure representing each student drawn on the chalkboard. When the students come in each day, they go to the chalkboard and chalk in a smile, or a frown, or whatever they feel. And they can change it later if their feelings change. Maybe I should put one on my front door to alert friends and save a lot of chitchat time.

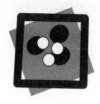

Taking a Break from Worry

Some of my friends think that I take troubles in life too lightly. Don't I realize, they insist, how harsh and cruel the world is? Maybe I don't want to. I know that I don't need to worry about the troubles that have temporarily slipped away from me. They won't have gone far.

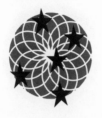

The Trials of Growing Up

Just when you think that at last you are growing up and facing cold reality, you may find that you've been fooled again!

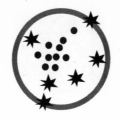

Beating the Odds

If you believe that you can beat the medical odds regarding your illness, you will increase your chances of doing so.

Finding a Balance

Walking the line between denial of your illness and preoccupation with it is not always easy; you can find a balance by facing the illness and doing all you can to effectively cope with it.

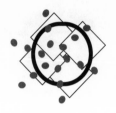

Contingent Plans

Making contingent plans, instead of promises you may not be able to keep, isn't expecting failure. It's setting realistic limits to help you protect yourself and feel more in control of your life.

Augment, Don't Substitute

When your biological family can't provide all the support you need, consider augmenting your care with friends and loved ones rather than substituting others for your family.

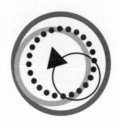

You Deserve Unconditional Love

A friend of mine came to me very upset, recently, because his father was not taking the preventive health measures that the son deemed appropriate. The son had decided to tell the father, "If you don't take better care of yourself, then don't expect me to be there for you when you get sick." I had to tell my friend that his ultimatum was unfair because it was based on conditional love. As children we expect unconditional love from our parents, but don't they also deserve that love?

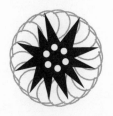

Personal or Conventional Priorities

In your search to reduce the demands on your daily life, it is helpful to categorize your priorities as either personal or conventional. The joy you derive from relationships and activities will be greater if you let your heart do the selecting rather than your head.

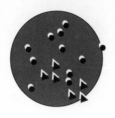

Good Physical Exercise

Exercise as much as you can physically, plus a bit more! A brisk walk, with arms swinging freely, is good for your body and helps keep you grounded in the "real" world.

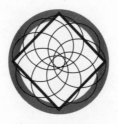

More Relaxation

Relax in a comfortable position several times a day. Unplug your telephone and lock the door if necessary. Say over and over to yourself, "Relax. No need to worry, no one to please. Rest and restore."

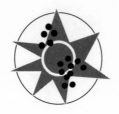

Expressing Your Love

Love the people you care for with all the passion you can muster. Love your mate, your family, and your friends. Express gratefulness to your caregivers. Express your love in as many ways as you can find, and then receive the love they have to give without fear of loss.

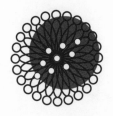

Helping Others Survive

When you can, help others who are experiencing similar conditions of survival. Don't just fight to stay alive for yourself, but for others, too. You are valuable and you make a difference.

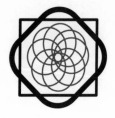

A Contented Spirit

Make sure you don't leave this life with any
words unspoken to the ones you love. Love
and be loved, and you cannot fail.

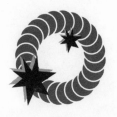

Asking for Help

One of the toughest lessons in life is accepting that it is necessary and okay to ask for help. You will have to eventually face it. No one person (even you) can do everything you may need.

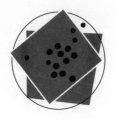

Identifying Stress

You can identify the signs of stress and anxiety within yourself. These include arguing with the one you need most, often over trivial matters. Sometimes, being stressed out will lead to a general feeling that it does not matter if your needs get met or not. More subtle signs include a creeping feeling of guilt for being a "burden" or some other such worry about being needy.

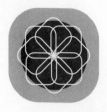

Communicating Needs

Each of us has a unique set of physical, emotional, and spiritual needs. Take the time to teach your caregivers about your hopes, fears, and plans for the future. Discuss openly what you need in order to feel content and cared for.

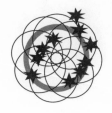

The Need for Control

Ideally, the family and loved ones closest to you should get together in person, by phone, or even by letter to assess and plan for your needs. You must be included in as many of these discussions as possible, so as to avoid feeling loss of control.

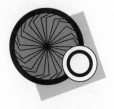

The Art of Caring

Caring is an act of attending to another's environment in a way that promotes inner and outer well-being. Caring is a therapeutic art. After all, medicine was first an art, then a science. Caregivers are fellow mortals with a good human understanding of the body, mind, and spirit. Caring is our most progressive adaptation to the conflicts and challenges in our lives.

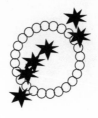

Trusting Your Knowledge

Trust in the knowledge that you do have the inner strength necessary to cope with whatever comes your way. Then give yourself permission to tap into that strength.

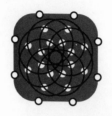

Giving to Yourself

Open yourself up to the compassion and love that exist within your heart. You would do all you could to nurture and comfort a dear friend who was afraid and hurting. So, allow yourself as much love and gentleness as you would give a dear friend.

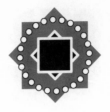

Your Tears As Love

Tears can be a gentle and loving way of ministering to yourself. Tears should be honored as tender drops of remembrance.

Doing Your Best

It is not appropriate to blame or to find fault with yourself. The truth is that you have always done your very best with the resources available to you.

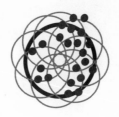

Letting Others Help

There are people who want to help you. Allow them the satisfaction of giving by allowing yourself to receive. Allow yourself the acknowledgment that you are not weak by receiving help, rather you are cared for and supported.

The Treasure of Loving

Your capacity for loving is your greatest treasure in life. Remember that love can flow in two directions—outward to the world and inward to yourself.

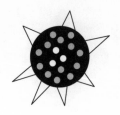

Your Daily Gifts

You are surrounded by gifts every living moment of every day. Let yourself feel appreciation for their presence in your life and take the time to acknowledge their splendor.

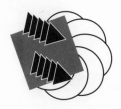

Five Life Commandments

Don't forget to take care of yourself while you are building on the past to make a brighter tomorrow. To help you do that, I want to share my Five Life Commandments:

1. Maintain honesty of communication.
2. Find joy in being and befriending.
3. Leave off possessing others.
4. Cling to visions of hope.
5. Get on with life.

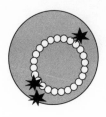

Obituaries Are Telling

Obituaries are often telling illustrations of our culture's attitudes about death, especially when they read, "So-and-so lost their struggle. . . ." I know that these people won every day of their lives as they lived triumphantly with stigmatizing and progressively debilitating illness.

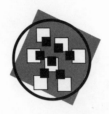

Living Is Not the Best Criteria for Success

I think we ought to pause for some serious thought before we blindly accept dying as a cultural criteria for failure, and by default, living as a success. I certainly know of more than one failure to live a full and happy life, and I have seen several deaths that were moments of profound truth and beauty.

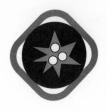

Blaming the Victim

There are those who feel sick children are "innocent." Does that mean sick adults are guilty? Does having AIDS, liver disease, cancer, etc., no matter how it came about, mean you brought it on yourself by smoking, drinking, having sex, sharing needles, etc.? Or are you just like all of us, learning life's lessons?

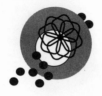

Giving In Rather Than Giving Up

People talk of "giving up" on life. It would be more positive to speak of letting go into the other side of life, or even of embracing death as graduating from life. We don't give up; we give in to a larger process.

Perspectives on Stress

Stress is largely related to our perspectives on death and illness. Examine your own "shoulds" about sickness and death. Appreciate that although you would prefer wellness and life, illness and death are not to be judged as wrong, or as failures.

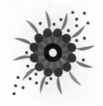

It Is Okay to Grieve

You won't like the way loss makes you feel. Although we can't control our emotions, we can control our response to them. Know that no matter how guilty you may feel over how the intensity of your feelings seems to make other people feel, you own those feelings; they are yours to experience and express freely. In other words, it is okay to grieve.

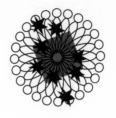

Loss May Feel Guilty

Don't let guilt for feelings about loss stop you from being in control of the emotions that you may deem to be negative. There are some priceless lessons to be learned about our own feelings toward life and death.

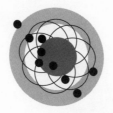

Learning from the Good
and the Bad

Acknowledge that you have done the best
with the resources you had to work with.
Also be prepared to acknowledge that you
can learn from any mistakes you feel you
may have made.

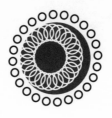

Be Here Now

If you only live with what was, you may miss the beautiful moments of what is. It is human to miss what you have loved and no longer have and to grieve for it, but try to be aware of the good things and the good people who are in your life now.

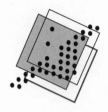

In Perfect Order

When it seems too overwhelming, take comfort in the knowledge that all is unfolding ac-
cording to a greater plan. Though this divine
plan may be beyond your ability to understand, trust that all is in perfect order.

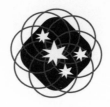

Share Each Moment

Though your heart is aching with the prospect of losing someone you dearly love, allow yourself to truly experience the precious moment with this person, and to share the gifts of love together.

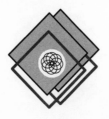

Looking To What You Now Have Versus What You Have Already Lost

Imagine your view is of the full moon rising between towering trees, with a nearby river lending its gentle caress to your ears. Now, stop counting the people you have lost to focus on the moments of life here and now.

Life Is Wonderful and Loss Is Undesirable

If life was a really awful human condition, why would we be upset over someone's loss of life, untimely or not? Life is wonderful! And it is sad to lose people to illness and death.

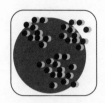

Life Is Not Meaningless

Death does not make life less meaningful, not even a little bit! In fact, it leads us to appreciate the gift of life with a recognition that while our bodies may be mortal our spirits are eternal.

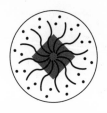

Discovering What You
Believe In and Cherish

In the Hebrew tradition, the word for prayer comes from a word which means "self-judgment." Prayer is looking into yourself, determining the meaning of life and death for you, finding out what is really of value to you, discovering what you really believe.

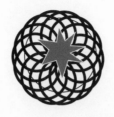

Read Your Heart and Help Yourself

Prayer is a tool for reading your own emotional state; use it to keep in touch with your feelings, to read your heart and help yourself. Pray by reminding yourself what really matters to you.

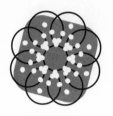

Prayer

Prayer is reaching higher, searching deeper, being truer to yourself and your purpose in life.

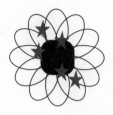

True Strength

Rather than using your prayers to ask that things become the way you want them to be, use your prayers to ask for the patience and courage to accept things the way they are. In acceptance and surrender you will find your true strength.

Perseverance and Surrender

We talk often about both perseverance and surrender. At first, I thought one precluded the other, but I am learning to cultivate both qualities and to recognize their harmonious natures.

Risk Being Real

Open your heart now to your loved one, and try not to hold back out of embarrassment or shyness. At a future time, you will find great comfort in knowing that nothing was left unsaid, that your loved one knew of your caring and your concerns, and that you were courageous and loving enough to risk being real.

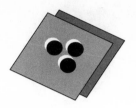

Celebrating Discoveries

You learned how to help me on your own. I don't know how, but I do know why. I celebrate your discoveries with you.

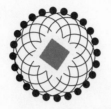

Gain Strength from Hard Times

Don't erase your memories of the times you held my hand at the doctor's office, or sat silently in the hospital room; rather, embrace these experiences and let them give you renewed strength and resolve.

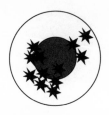

The Simple Things

Some days it is just the simple things you do that mean so much, like encouraging me to eat when I am depressed or otherwise lack an appetite. These are the times I quietly acknowledge to myself that your caring will always be there.

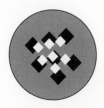

Don't Dissuade Me, Just Listen

When I feel like giving up, when I want to die and get it all over with, you don't dissuade me from my apprehensions. You just listen and do your best to understand my fears.

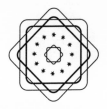

Remind Me of My Value

When I question the value of my continued existence, you remind me that I am a valuable person who enhances your life and the lives of those who love me.

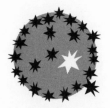

In the Heart They Remain

When you look to the night sky and wonder, Where have they gone? place your hands over your heart space and know they are right here.

About the Author

In 1983 Lon Nungesser was diagnosed with terminal cancer and given three months to live. He designed his own medical treatment, and his cancer went into remission in 1985. With the support of Dr. Philip Zimbardo, Nungesser worked on psychosocial intervention for people with AIDS at the psychology department of Stanford University. In addition to *Axioms for Survivors,* he has published *Epidemic of Courage: Facing AIDS in America* and *Notes On Living Until We Say Goodbye: A Personal Guide.* Nungesser is now in his ninth year of survival since his "terminal" diagnosis.

The University of Michigan at Ann Arbor has acquired Nungesser's life works, unpublished autobiography, and photo albums in a special collection called "The Nungesser Papers: Hope for Humanity." Proceeds from

Nungesser's previous publications have been donated by him to a special fund established by the university's regents to fund research on the link between social oppression and physical disease, and reformations in American medicine. The fund is called The Lonnie Gene Nungesser Research Fund.

For further information about the work, life, and times of Lon Nungesser, contact The Harlan Hatcher Graduate Library, The Department of Rare Books and Special Collections, University of Michigan at Ann Arbor, Ann Arbor, Michigan 48109-1205.